Smoothie Cookbook

Simple and Detail Recipes for Beginners to Make Delicious and Healthy Smoothie

Mendocino Bruner

DISCAIMER

The content, writing, images, photos, descriptions and information contained in this book are for general guidance and are intended for informational purposes only for the readers. The author has narrated his cooking and research experiences in this book by observing and evaluating relevant facts and figures. The author is not a registered dietitian and nutritional information in this book should only be used as a general guideline. Statements in this book have not been evaluated or approved by any regulatory authority.

The author has tried to provide all the information related to the ingredients, foods, and products, however, when certain ingredients get mixed, they may create some kind of cross-reaction which may cause allergy among some people.

There may be products that will not be gluten-free and may contain ingredients that may cause a reaction. These products may include but are limited to, eggs, dairy, wheat, nuts, coconut, flour, soy, cocoa, milk, sugar, and other products.

These may cause allergic reactions in some people due to cross-contamination from allergen-causing products.

The readers and purchasers of this book understand and consent that there may be ingredients in the foods which may contain certain allergens and the readers and purchasers hereby disclaimer the author of this book from all liabilities related to allergic and cross food reactions.

The information provided in this book must not be taken as an alternative to any advice by a doctor, physician, dietitian or health care specialist. The readers should not use the information given in this book for diagnosing an illness or other health-related problems. Furthermore, the readers also should not discontinue professional medical or healthcare advice because of something they have read in this book. The content and information provided in this book do not create any kind of professional relationship between the reader and the author of this book.

This book in no way provides any warranty, express or implied, towards the content of recipes contained in this book.

It is the reader's responsibility to determine the value and quality of any recipe or instructions provided for food preparation and to determine the nutritional value if any, and safety of the preparation instructions. Therefore, the author of this book is not responsible for the outcome of any recipe that a reader may try from this book. The readers of this book may not always have the same results due to variations in ingredients, humidity, altitude, cooking temperatures, errors, omissions, or individual cooking abilities.

The images and photos contained in this book may have been used for representational, informative and information purposes and may not be the exact match of the accompanying recipes. These images and photos provide the author's impression of how a particular recipe might look after it has been cooked, made or completed and the images and photos should only be relied upon for the purpose of reference and not actual finished products, recipes or foods.

By purchasing this book, readers hereby acknowledge that they are going to rely on any information provided in the book 'as-is' and must not use this information to form any final conclusion, whether the information is in the form of description, recipe, or ingredient.

Readers agree that they will consult a physician, dietitian or professional healthcare specialist before using and relying on any data, information, or suggestion described in this book. Readers agree to accept all risks of relying upon and using any of the information presented in this book. Readers also agree to hold harmless the author, editor, publisher, affiliates, team, and staff members or anyone associated with this book from and against any damages, lawsuits, costs, claims, expenses including any legal fees, medical fees, or insurance fees resulting from the application of any of the information provided by this book. Any reliance readers make on any information presented in this book is at their sole discretion and risk. The author of this book hereby disclaims any liability in connection with the use of any information presented in this book.

Table of Contents

Blueberry Lime Smoothie

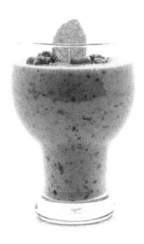

Preparation time: 1-2 minutes
Blending time: 3 minutes
Servings: 2

Ingredients

- 1 cup greek yogurt
- 2 tbsp lime juice

- 1 cup ice cubes
- 1 tsp lime zest
- 1 cup frozen blueberries
- 2 celery stalks

Instructions

- Blend Greek yogurt, lime juice, lime zest, frozen blueberries, celery stalks, and ice cubes in a blender, for approximately 3 minutes.

Blueberry-Watermelon Smoothie

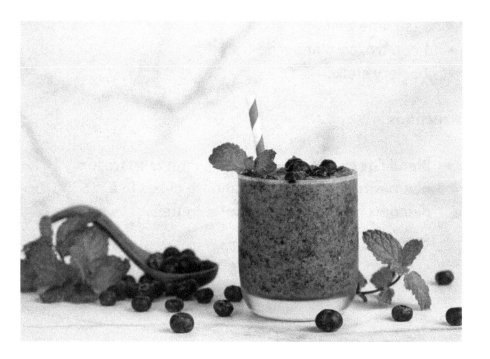

Preparation time: 1-2 minutes
Blending time: 2 minutes
Servings: 2

Ingredients

- 1 cup watermelon scoops
- 1 cup coconut water
- 12 mint leaves
- ¼ tsp cinnamon
- 1 cup ice cubes
- 1 tbsp chia seeds
- 1 cup frozen blueberries

Instructions
- Intermingle these healthy ingredients i.e. watermelon, coconut water, mint leaves, cinnamon, ice cubes, and chia seeds in a blender for 2 minutes and serve.

Fresh fig Green Smoothie

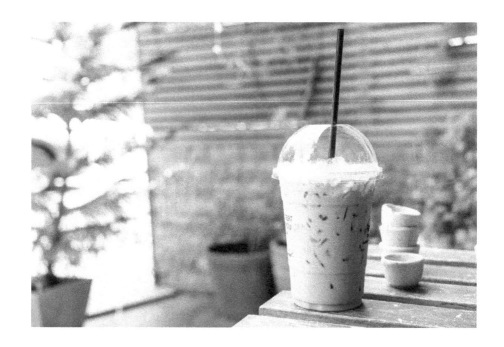

Preparation time: 1-2 minutes
Blending time: 2 minutes
Servings: 2

Ingredients

- 1 cup avocados
- ½ cup fresh figs with its skin removed
- 1 cup baby spinach leaves
- 1 cup hemp milk
- 1 cup ice cubes
- 1 tbsp cashew nuts

Instructions

- Combine and blend all these ingredients in a blender for approximately 2 minutes.

Blackberry lemon smoothie

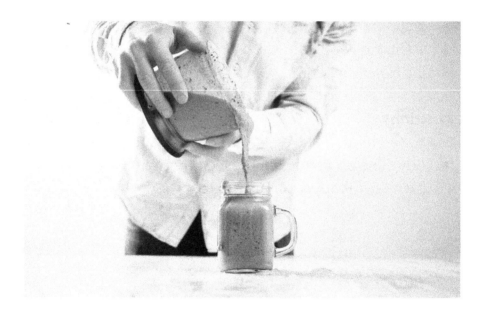

Preparation time: 1-2 minutes
Blending time: 3 minutes
Servings: 2

Ingredients

- 1 tbsp collagen protein powder
- 1 cup ice cubes
- 1 cup frozen blackberries
- 1 tsp fresh lemon zest
- ½ cup frozen raspberries
- 2 tbsp lemon juice
- 1 tbsp flax seeds
- 1 cup heavy cream (unsweetened)

Instructions

- Blend these ingredients very well until they become smooth and single textured.

Strawberry smoothie

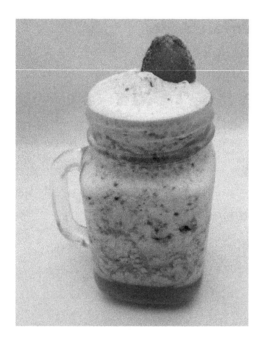

Preparation time: 1-2 minutes
Blending time: 3 minutes
Servings: 2

Ingredients

- 1 cup heavy cream
- ½ cup frozen strawberries
- ½ cup frozen blueberries
- ½ cup frozen cranberries
- ½ cup frozen raspberries
- 1 tbsp chia seeds
- ¼ tsp cinnamon
- 1 tsp pistachio butter

Instructions

- Put heavy cream, frozen strawberries, blueberries, cranberries, raspberries, ice, chia seeds, cinnamon, and pistachio butter in the blender. Swirl until smooth and creamy.

Cucumber and Olive Smoothie

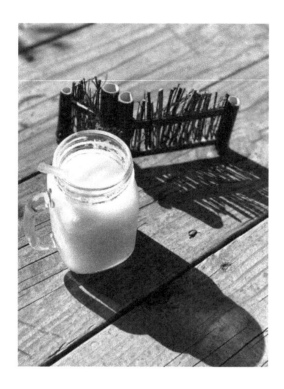

Preparation time: 1-2 minutes
Blending time: 2 minutes
Servings: 2

Ingredients

- 2 cups diced cucumbers
- ½ cup parsley
- ½ cup celery
- ½ cup green olives
- 1 cup ice cubes
- ½ cup black olives
- 1 cup greek yogurt
- 1 tsp coconut oil
- 1 tsp chia seeds

Instructions

- Swirl cucumbers, parsley, black olives, ice cubes, green olives, celery, parsley, greek yogurt, coconut oil, and chia seeds in a blender until thick and creamy.

Rich Roman Lettuce Smoothie

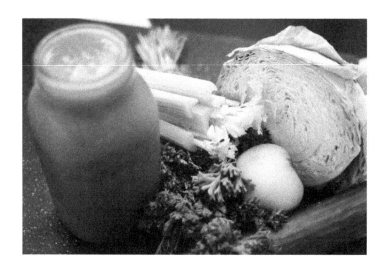

Preparation time: 1-2 minutes
Blending time: 2 minutes
Servings: 2

Ingredients

- 2 cups Roman lettuce
- 1 cup baby spinach
- 1 tbsp lime juice
- 1 tbsp lemon juice
- 1 cup almond milk
- 1 cup ice

Instructions

- Jumble these ingredients in the blender first on pulse mode and then on juicer mode until they are well combined and smooth.

Kiwi-Avocado Smoothie

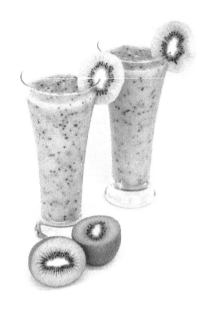

Preparation time: 1-2 minutes
Blending time: 2 minutes
Servings: 2

Ingredients

- 2 cups kiwi-diced
- 1 cup ice cubes
- 1 cup avocado slices
- 1 cup kale leaves
- ½ tsp spirulina powder
- 2 tbsp lemon juice
- 1 cup unsweetened coconut milk

Instructions

- Mix kiwi, ice cubes, avocado slices, kale leaves, spirulina powder, lemon juice, and unsweetened coconut milk in a blender until a creamy thick consistency is achieved.

Green asparagus smoothie

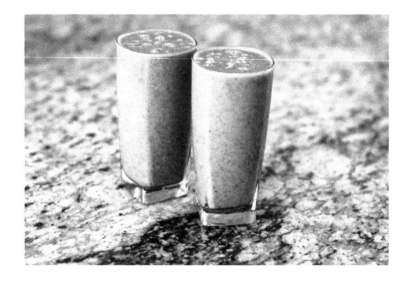

Preparation time: 1-2 minutes
Blending time: 2 minutes
Servings: 2

Ingredients

- ½ cup asparagus
- 1 cup avocados
- 1 cup diced cucumbers
- 12 mint leaves
- 1 cup coconut water
- 1 tbsp collagen
- ½ tsp sea salt

Instructions

- Intermingle asparagus, avocados, diced cucumbers, mint leaves, coconut water, collagen, ice cubes, and sea salt, in a blender to achieve a creamy texture.

Cherry coconut smoothie

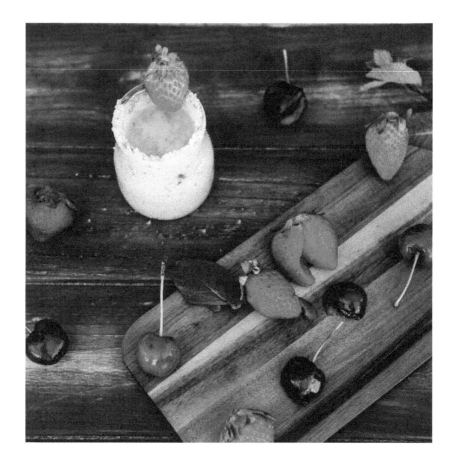

Preparation time: 1-2 minutes
Blending time: 2 minutes
Servings:

Ingredients

- 1 cup frozen cherries
- 2 tbsp shredded coconut
- 1 cup coconut water
- Few drops of liquid monk fruit
- 1 tbsp hemp seeds
- 1 tbsp collagen powder
- Few ice cubes

Instructions

- Mix these ingredients in a blender until it reaches a thick consistent uniform mixture.

Peach-plum smoothie

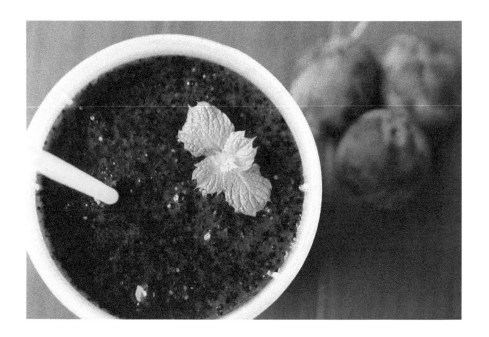

Preparation time: 1-2 minutes
Blending time: 2 minutes
Servings: 2

Ingredients

- 1 cup diced peaches
- 1 cup plum cubes
- 1 cup watermelon cubes
- 2 tbsp lemon juice
- 12 mint leaves
- 1 tbsp flaxseeds
- 1 cup simple ice water
- Few ice cubes

Instructions

- All the ingredients including peaches, plums, watermelon, lemon juice, mint leaves, flaxseeds, and ice water should be blended to form a thick smoothie.

Three-Nut smoothie

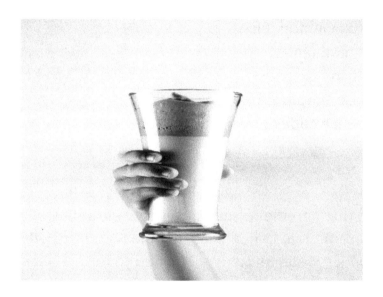

Preparation time: 1-2 minutes
Blending time: 2 minutes
Servings: 2

Ingredients

- ½ cup walnuts
- ¼ cup cashews
- ½ cup hazelnuts
- ¼ tsp vanilla extract
- 1 cup heavy coconut cream (unsweetened)
- 1 tsp almond butter
- 1 tbsp erythritol
- Few ice cubes

Instructions

- Put all these entities in the blender and keep on blending until a uniform smoothie is formed with thickened consistency.

Lemon Tomato Smoothie

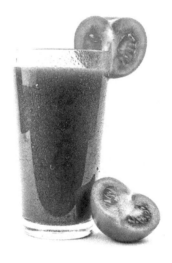

Preparation time: 1-2 minutes
Blending time: 2 minutes
Servings: 2

Ingredients

- 1 ½ cup diced tomatoes
- 1 cup cabbage
- 3 tbsp lemon juice
- 1 cup iced water
- 10-12 mint leaves
- ¼ tsp sea salt
- 1 cup ice cubes

Instructions

- Mix all of these ingredients in a blender until smooth.

Cantaloupe Basil Smoothie

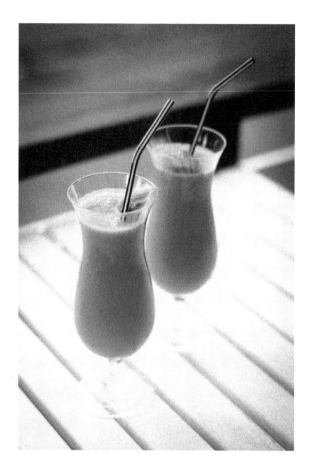

Preparation time: 1-2 minutes
Blending time: 2 minutes
Servings: 2

Ingredients

- 1 cup cantaloupe cubes
- 1 cup basil leaves
- 4 celery stalks
- 1 cup ice cubes
- 1 cup fresh orange juice
- 1 tsp pistachios
- 1 tsp chia seeds

Instructions

- In the blender, add cantaloupe, basil leaves, celery stalks, orange juice, ice cubes, pistachios, and chia seeds and swirl until well combined.

Turmeric Pineapple Swirl Smoothie

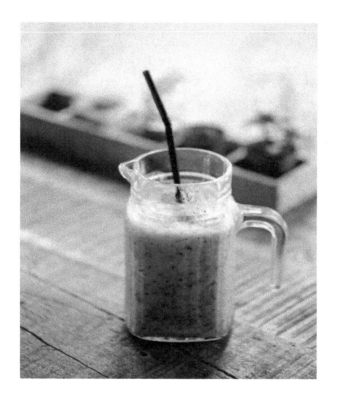

Preparation time: 1-2 minutes
Blending time: 2 minutes
Servings: 2

Ingredients

- 1 ½ cup pineapple cubes
- 1 cup cabbage
- ½ tsp turmeric
- ¼ cup fresh mint
- 1 tbsp protein powder of your choice
- 1 cup iced water

Instructions

- Mix all these ingredients in a blender and blend until creamy fluffy texture is achieved.

Raspberry Vanilla Smoothie

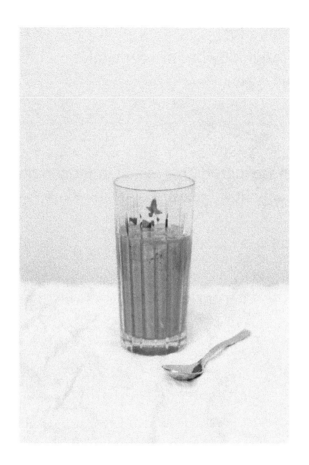

Preparation time: 1-2 minutes
Blending time: 2 minutes
Servings: 2

Ingredients

- 2 cups frozen raspberries
- 1 cup heavy coconut cream (unsweetened)
- ¼ cup almonds
- ½ cup almond milk
- ½ tsp vanilla essence
- 2 tsp chia seeds

Instructions

- Blend all of these ingredients until smooth and uniform.

Berry Walnut Smoothie

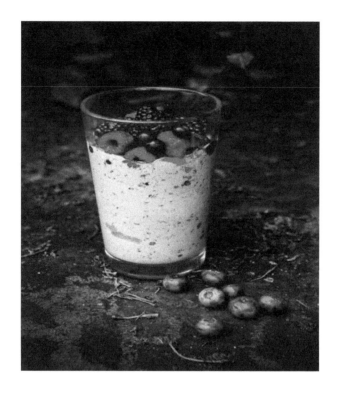

Preparation time: 1-2 minutes
Blending time: 2 minutes
Servings: 2

Ingredients

- 1 cup frozen raspberries
- 1 cup frozen cranberries
- 1 cup frozen strawberries
- ½ cup walnuts
- 1 tsp walnut butter
- 1 cup unsweetened heavy cream
- 1 tsp stevia

Instructions

- Simply put all these ingredients in a blender and swirl them until they are uni textured.

Strawberry Cream Smoothie

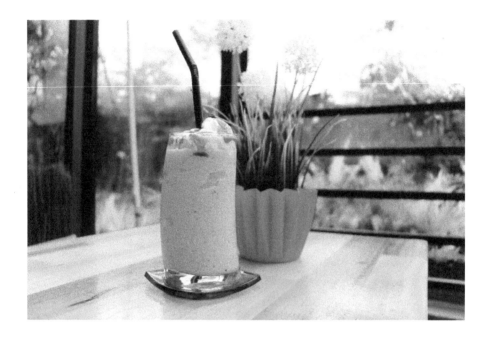

Preparation time: 1-2 minutes
Blending time: 2 minutes
Servings: 2

Ingredients

- 2 cups frozen strawberries
- ¼ cup Macadamia Nut milk
- ½ cup unsweetened heavy cream
- ½ tsp erythritol
- ½ cup dairy-free cream cheese
- Few ice cubes

Instructions

- Fill the blending jar with these mentioned substances and blend to get a creamy smoothie.

Starfruit berry mix smoothie

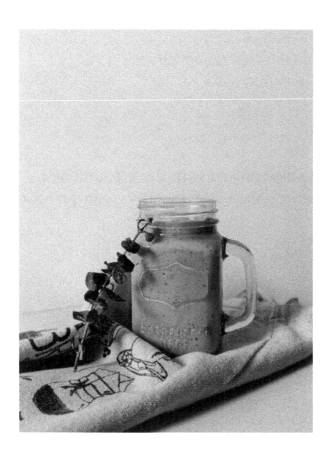

Preparation time: 1-2 minutes
Blending time: 2 minutes
Servings: 2

Ingredients

- 1 cup starfruit
- 1 cup frozen blueberries
- 1 cup frozen blackberries
- ½ cup cherries
- 1 cup coconut water
- 1 tsp keto base powder

Instructions

- Blend all of these ingredients to get a thick smoothie.

Green Cantaloupe Smoothie

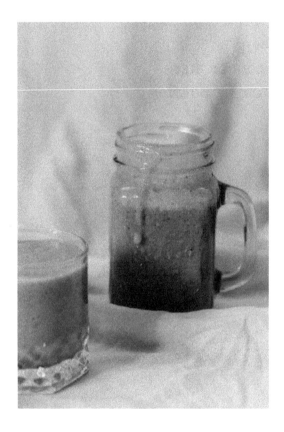

Preparation time: 1-2 minutes
Blending time: 2 minutes
Servings: 2

Ingredients

- 2 cups of Cantaloupe
- 2 cups of spinach
- 1 tsp almond butter
- 1 cup unsweetened heavy cream
- Few ice cubes

Instructions

- Combine ice, spinach, almond butter, cantaloupe, and heavy cream in the blender. Blend on high speed until it is smooth. Pour in the glasses and serve.

Peach Mojito Smoothie

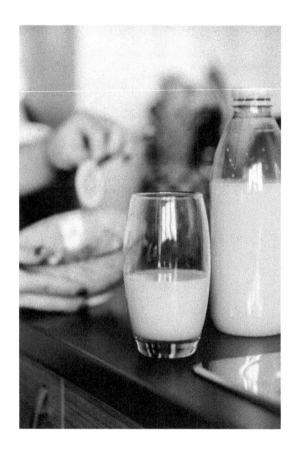

Preparation time: 1-2 minutes
Blending time: 2 minutes
Servings: 2

Ingredients

- 2 cups of peaches-thick slices
- 1 cup hemp milk
- 1 cup ice cubes
- 2 tbsp lime juice
- 12 mint leaves

Instructions

- In the blender, add all of these ingredients and mix until all the constituents are thoroughly mixed.
- Stream the smoothie in the glasses and serve.

Celery rich Smoothie

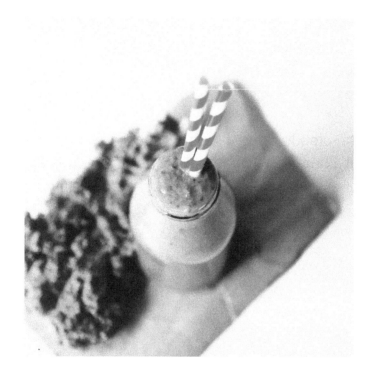

Preparation time: 1-2 minutes
Blending time: 2 minutes
Servings: 2

Ingredients

- 2 cups celery
- 1 cup baby spinach
- ½ cup kale
- ½ cup zucchini
- 1 cup greek yogurt
- ½ tbsp chia seeds
- Few ice cubes

Instructions

- Put all these elements in the blender and blend at high speed to get them equally mixed.

Cabbage Margarita Smoothie

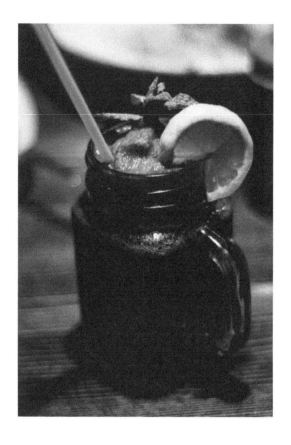

Preparation time: 1-2 minutes
Blending time: 2 minutes
Servings: 2

Ingredients

- 2 cups cabbage
- 1 cup mint
- ½ tsp mint extract
- ½ tsp coconut oil
- 1 cup heavy cream (unsweetened)
- 1 tbsp stevia

Instructions

- At high speed blend all of these ingredients and pour them into the glasses and present.

Pina-Kale Smoothie

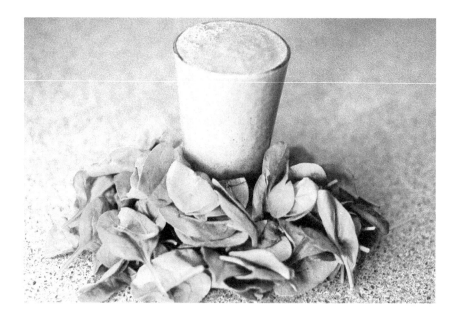

Preparation time: 1-2 minutes
Blending time: 2 minutes
Servings: 2

Ingredients

- 2 cups of pineapple cubes
- 1 ½ cup of kale
- Stevia (according to taste)
- 1 cup ice cubes
- 4 lettuce leaves
- 1 tsp ketone base powder of your choice
- 1 cup almond milk

Instructions

- Put all these ingredients in the blender at high speed also at pulse mode to crush all the ice. Serve in glass mugs.

Almond Peach Smoothie

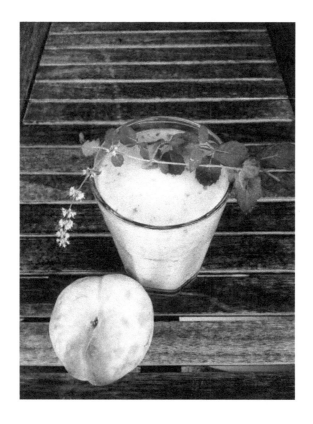

Preparation time: 1-2 minutes
Blending time: 2 minutes
Servings: 2

Ingredients

- ½ cup almonds
- 1 cup almond milk
- 2 cups peach cubes
- Stevia (according to desired sweetness)
- ½ tsp cinnamon powder

Instructions

- Whirl almonds, peaches, ice cubes, stevia, and cinnamon powder on high speed in the blender and present by pouring it in your favorite glasses.

Avocado Flaxseed smoothie

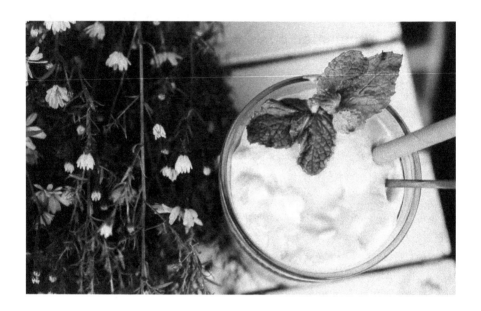

Preparation time: 1-2 minutes
Blending time: 2 minutes
Servings: 2

Ingredients

- 2 cups of sliced or diced avocados
- 1 cup Bok choy
- 1 tbsp flaxseeds
- 1 cup unsweetened coconut cream
- Few ice cubes
- ¼ cup of cashew milk
- 1 tbsp collagen powder

Instructions

- Whirl all of these substances in the blender at high speed and pulse mode until a well-combined smoothie is formed.

Zucchini Green Smoothie

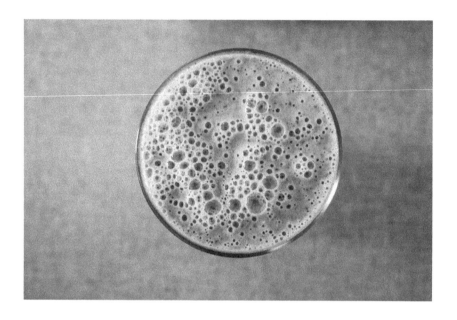

Preparation time: 1-2 minutes
Blending time: 2 minutes
Servings: 2

Ingredients

- 1 ½ cup zucchini
- 1 cup Bok Choy
- 12 mint leaves
- ½ cup spinach
- 1 cup ice cubes
- 1 cup normal mineral water

Instructions

- Put all of these constituents of smoothie in the blender and mix at high speed until well combined.

Spinach Cream Smoothie

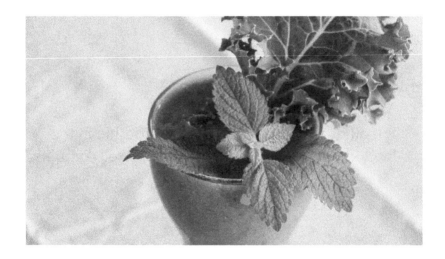

Preparation time: 1-2 minutes
Blending time: 2 minutes
Servings: 2

Ingredients

- 2 cups of spinach
- 2 tbsp lemon juice
- ½ cup cream cheese (dairy-free)
- 1 cup unsweetened heavy cream
- 1 cup celery
- Stevia (according to your desired sweetness)
- Few ice cubes

Instructions

- Put all these mentioned ingredients in the blender and blend to form a creamy texture mixture.

Raspberry Lemonade Smoothie

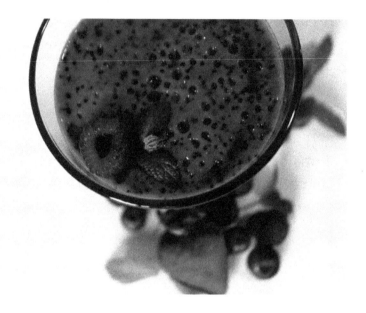

Preparation time: 1-2 minutes
Blending time: 2 minutes
Servings: 2

Ingredients

- 2 cups of frozen raspberries
- 2 tbsp lemon juice
- 1 tbsp lime juice
- ½ green apple
- 12 leaves of mint
- Few ice cubes
- 1 cup iced water
- 2 tsp monk fruit liquid

Instructions

- To make this yummy healthy detox swirl together all these ingredients at high speed in the blender. When all are thoroughly mixed pour them in the glass and serve.

Coffee Spirulina Smoothie

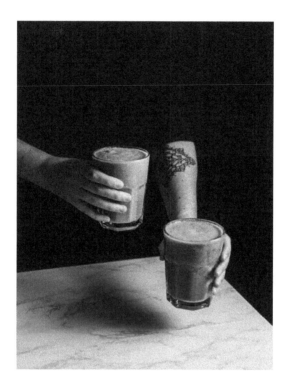

Preparation time: 1-2 minutes
Blending time: 2 minutes
Servings: 2

Ingredients

- 1 tbsp coffee-flavored protein powder
- 2 tbsp monk fruit liquid
- 1 tbsp spirulina powder
- 1 tsp almond butter
- Unsweetened dairy-free cream
- ½ tsp unsweetened cocoa
- Few ice cubes

Instructions

- Blend all of these ingredients in the blender until creamy and smooth. You can variate your ingredient choice i.e. you can add berries.

Salty Cocoa Smoothie

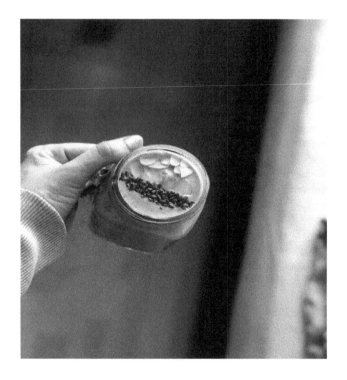

Preparation time: 1-2 minutes
Blending time: 2 minutes
Servings: 2

Ingredients

- 1 tsp unsweetened cocoa powder
- ½ tsp sea salt
- 1 cup avocados
- 1 cup dairy-free milk
- 1 tbsp protein powder
- Few ice cubes

Instructions

- Blend all these constituents to form a thick smoothie. Pour in the glass or smoothie jars and enjoy.

Choco-Peanut Butter Smoothie

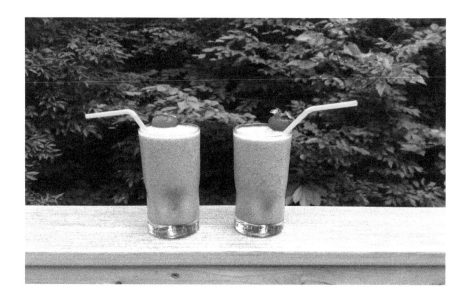

Preparation time: 1-2 minutes
Blending time: 2 minutes
Servings: 2

Ingredients

- 1 tsp unsweetened cocoa
- 1 cup dairy-free coconut cream
- ½ cup cashew nuts
- 1 cup walnuts
- Stevia (as per taste)
- Few ice cubes
- ½ cup shredded coconut
- 1 tbsp peanut butter

Instructions

- In a mixer or a blender, blend all of these mentioned ingredients to make this delicious mouth-watering smoothie.

Pink Smoothie

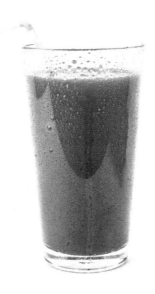

Preparation time: 1-2 minutes
Blending time: 2 minutes
Servings: 2

Ingredients

- 1 tbsp dragon fruit powder
- 1 cup frozen cranberries
- 1 cup fresh diced dragon fruit
- 1 tbsp chia seeds
- 1 tbsp exogenous ketone base
- Ice cubes

Instructions

- At high speed, blend dragon fruit, cranberries, chia seeds, ketone base, dragonfruit powder, and ice cubes. Pour it in glasses and serve.

Mint Green Smoothie

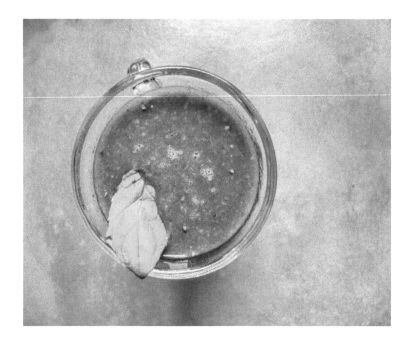

Preparation time: 1-2 minutes
Blending time: 2 minutes
Servings: 2

Ingredients

- 1 cup mint leaves
- 1 cup avocados
- 1 cup basil
- ½ cup lemon juice
- 1 cup hemp milk
- Few ice cubes

Instructions

- Put all of these ingredients in the blender and mix until well combined.

Healthy Breakfast Oat Smoothie

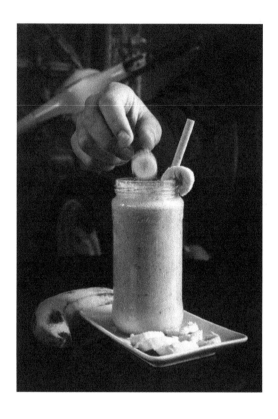

Preparation time: 1-2 minutes
Blending time: 2 minutes
Servings: 2

Ingredients

- 1 tbsp oat powder
- 2 cups avocados
- ½ ripe banana
- 1 tsp hemp seeds
- 1 cup ice cubes
- ½ cup coconut dairy-free cream

Instructions

- Add these mentioned ingredients to the blender and swirl them together for 1 or 2 minutes at pulse and blender mode.

Almond Milk Strawberry Smoothie

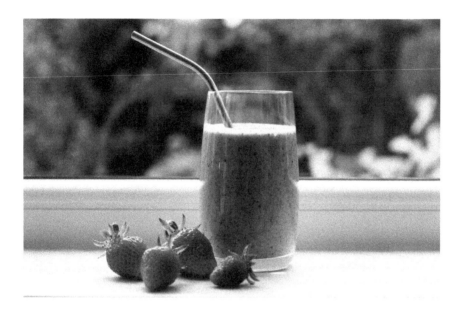

Preparation time: 1-2 minutes
Blending time: 2 minutes
Servings: 2

Ingredients

- 1 tbsp almond butter
- 1 cup almond milk
- 1 ½ cup frozen strawberries
- ½ cup almonds (soaked overnight & peeled)
- Stevia (as per your taste)
- 1 tbsp collagen powder
- Few ice cubes

Instructions

- Whirl all these ingredients in the blender until smooth and fluffy.

Strawberry Nut Smoothie

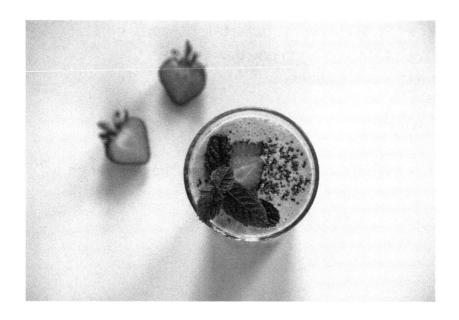

Preparation time: 1-2 minutes
Blending time: 2 minutes
Servings: 2

Ingredients

- ½ cup walnuts
- ½ cup hazelnuts
- ½ cup cashews
- 2 cups frozen strawberries
- 1 cup coconut cream (dairy-free)
- 1 tsp walnut butter
- Monk fruit liquid (as per your taste)
- Few ice cubes

Instructions

- Blend walnuts, hazelnuts, cashews, frozen strawberries, coconut cream, walnut butter, and monk fruit liquid to get a thick consistency protein smoothie.

Plain Peanut butter Smoothie

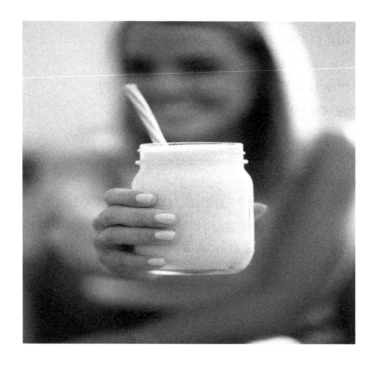

Preparation time: 1-2 minutes
Blending time: 2 minutes
Servings: 2

Ingredients

- 1 tbsp peanut butter
- 1 tbsp exogenous ketone base
- 1 tsp chia seeds
- ½ cup almond milk
- ½ cup shredded coconut
- ¼ tsp cinnamon
- ¼ tsp cardamom powder
- Few ice cubes

Instructions

- Add the following entities in the juicer and blend until everything is mixed up.

Blueberry Keto Smoothie

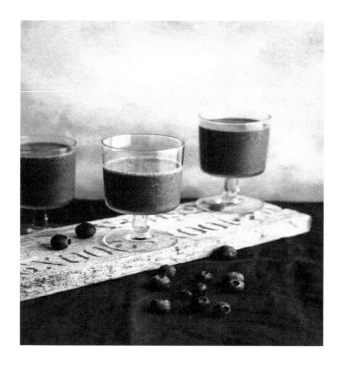

Preparation time: 1-2 minutes
Blending time: 2 minutes
Servings: 2

Ingredients

- 2 cups frozen blueberries
- ½ cup almond powder
- ½ cup pistachio powder
- ½ cup walnut powder
- 1 tsp coconut oil
- Few ice cubes
- 1 cup heavy cream (unsweetened & dairy-free)

Instructions

- Combine all of the following ingredients in the blender and serve it

Berry Swirl Smoothie

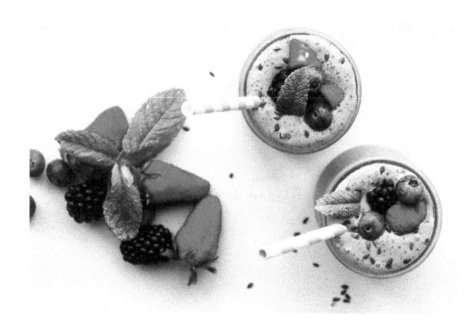

Preparation time: 1-2 minutes
Blending time: 2 minutes
Servings: 2

Ingredients

- 1 cup frozen blackberries
- ½ cup frozen raspberries
- ½ cup frozen blueberries
- 2-3 dates (seed removed)
- ½ cup almond milk
- Stevia (as per your taste)
- Few ice cubes
- ½ cup heavy cream (unsweetened)

Instructions

- Put all of these ingredients in the blender except heavy cream and blend. Pour it into glasses when it is well mixed.
- Pour heavy cream in the glasses and swirl with one or two strokes using a spoon or a straw.

Avocado Lemon Smoothie

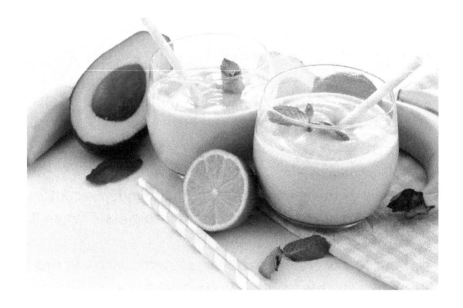

Preparation time: 1-2 minutes
Blending time: 2 minutes
Servings: 2

Ingredients

- 2 ½ cup avocados
- 2 tbsp lemon juice
- 2 tbsp lime juice
- Few ice cubes
- Monk fruit liquid(as per taste)
- 1 tsp lime & lemon zest
- 1 cup hemp milk

Instructions

- Blend all of these ingredients until well combined. Stream it into the glasses and serve with sprinkled lemon zest.

Chocolate Smoothie

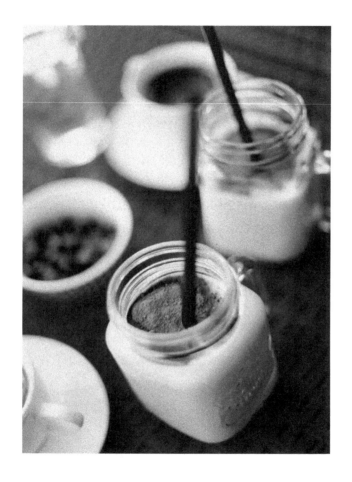

Preparation time: 1-2 minutes
Blending time: 2 minutes
Servings: 2

Ingredients

- ½ cup hemp milk
- 1 tsp exogenous ketone base
- 1 tsp cocoa (unsweetened)
- ½ cup heavy cream
- 1 tsp walnut butter
- Few ice cubes

Instructions

- To make the smoothie whirl all the above-written ingredients in the blender.

Spinach & Basil Smoothie

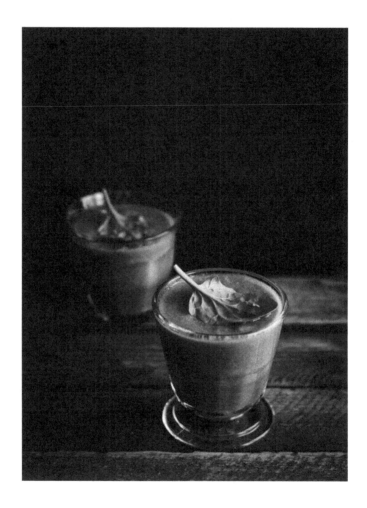

Preparation time: 1-2 minutes
Blending time: 2 minutes
Servings: 2

Ingredients

- 2 cups baby spinach leaves
- 2 cups of basil leaves
- ¼ cup stevia
- ½ cup lettuce
- ½ cup iced water
- Few ice cubes
- 1 tsp exogenous ketone base

Instructions

- For making this yummy smoothie, blend all of these written ingredients in the juicer. Serve with basil leaves on top.

Choco-berry Smoothie

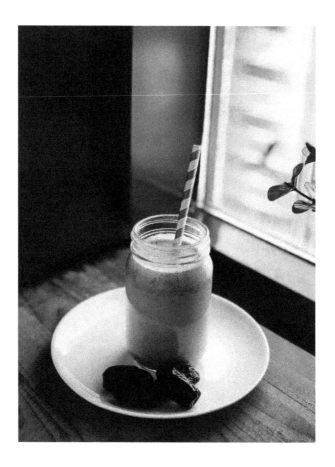

Preparation time: 1-2 minutes
Blending time: 2 minutes
Servings: 2

Ingredients

- 1 tsp unsweetened cocoa
- 1 tsp any chocolate-flavored protein powder
- 1 cup frozen raspberries
- 1 cup frozen strawberries
- 1 tsp hazelnut butter
- 1 tsp stevia
- 1 cup heavy dairy-free unsweetened cream

Instructions

- In the blending machine, add all of the above-written ingredients and keep it on the blending mode until a smooth consistency is achieved.

Spinach Raspberry Smoothie

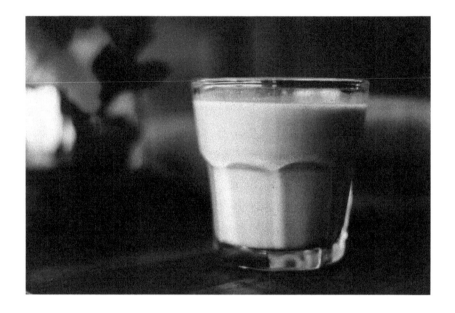

Preparation time: 1-2 minutes
Blending time: 2 minutes
Servings: 2

Ingredients

- 2 cups of spinach
- 1 cup of raspberries
- 2 tbsp lime juice
- Few ice cubes
- Ice cold water

Instructions

- Put all of the following constituents in a blender and keep on blending until a uni-textured smoothie is achieved.

Dragon fruit berry Smoothie

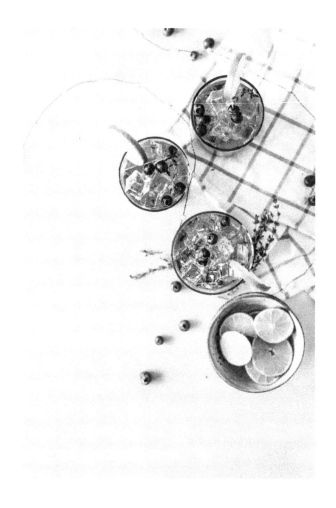

Preparation: 1-2 minutes
Blending time: 2 minutes
Servings: 2

Ingredients

- 1 cup dragon fruits
- 1 cup frozen strawberries
- 1 cup frozen raspberries
- ½ cup lemon juice
- ½ cup iced water
- Few ice cubes

Instructions

- In the electric blending machine, mix all of these ingredients, in blending mode to make the smoothie.

Cucumber green Smoothie

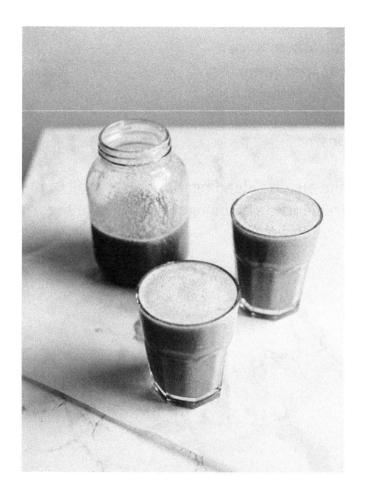

Preparation time: 1-2 minutes
Blending time: 2 minutes
Servings: 2

Ingredients

- 2 cups diced cucumbers
- 1 cup pear
- 1 cup celery
- 12 mint leaves
- 1 tsp lemon zest
- 2 tsp lime juice
- 1 cup ice cubes
- 1 cup iced water

Instructions

- Whirl these rich green ingredients in the blender very well, serve in milkshake jars.

Lemon ginger smoothie

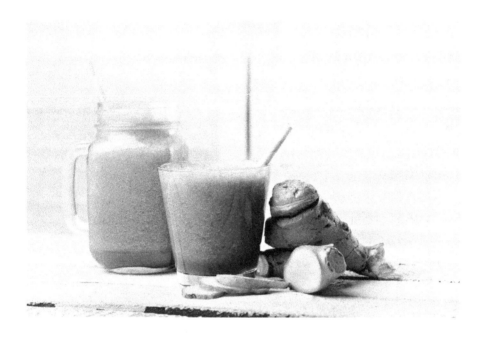

Preparation time: 1-2 minutes
Blending time: 2 minutes
Servings: 2

Ingredients

- 3 tbsp lemon juice
- 1 tsp orange zest
- 4-5 ginger slices
- 1 tsp collagen
- ½ cup spinach
- 1 cup avocados
- Ice cubes (as much needed)
- Pineapple juice (sugar-free)

Instructions

- Add all of these ingredients to the mixer and keep on blending till all the entities are well jumbled.

Green Pineapple Smoothie

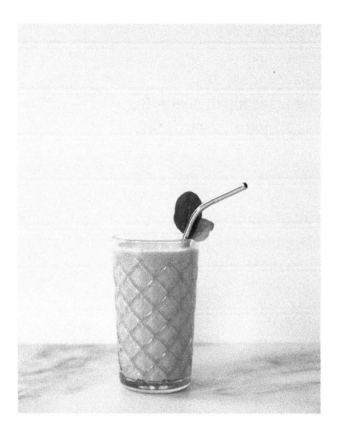

Preparation time: 1-2 minutes
Blending time: 2 minutes
Servings: 2

Ingredients

- 1 cup pears
- 2 cups of pineapple
- 1 cup avocado
- ½ cup coconut milk (dairy-free)
- ½ cup pistachios
- Few ice cubes

Instructions

- Whirl the following ingredients in the blender. Put few pineapple slices in the glass and pour the smoothie above it.

Avocado Chocolate Smoothie

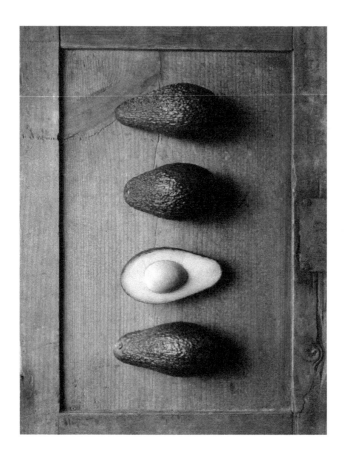

Preparation time: 1-2 minutes
Blending time: 2 minutes
Servings; 2

Ingredients

- 2 cups avocado
- 1 tsp unsweetened cocoa
- 1 tsp hazelnut butter
- 1 tsp hazelnuts
- Few ice cubes
- ½ cup coconut milk

Instructions

- Add these ingredients to the blender and keep on jumbling at blending mode until thoroughly mixed.

Avocados And Banana Smoothie

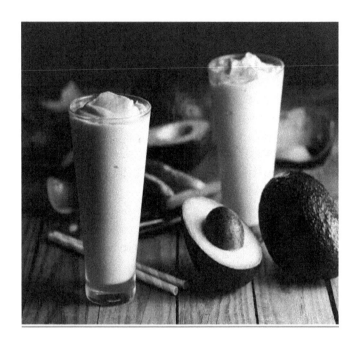

Preparation time: 1-2 minutes
Blending time: 2 minutes
Servings: 2

Ingredients

- 4 ripe bananas
- 3 cups of coconut water
- 2 cups of mashed avocados
- 2 tablespoons of honey
- 6 ice cubes
- 2-4. Chopped mint leaves

Instructions

- Take a blender add all the ingredients, then blend it for 5-6 minutes until smooth creamy mixture formed

BlueBerry Smoothie

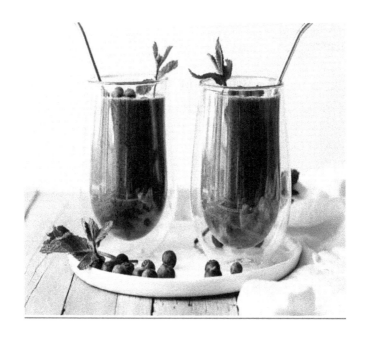

Preparation time: 1-2 minutes
Blending time: 2 minutes
Servings: 2

Ingredients

- 2 frozen bananas
- 1 cup of unsweetened almond milk
- 3 cups of wild blueberries
- 1 teaspoon of pumpkin seeds
- 1 teaspoon of maple syrup
- 1 teaspoon of ripe avocado

Instructions

- Take a blender add all the ingredients into a blender one by one then blend it until smooth creamy mixture formed

Special Mediterranean Tropical Smoothie

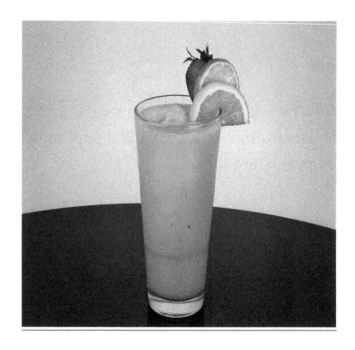

Preparation time: 1-2 minutes
Blending time: 2 minutes
Servings: 2

Ingredients

- 2 cups of orange pulp
- 1 tablespoon of lemon juice
- 1 cup of frozen strawberries
- 1 cup of frozen bananas
- 1 teaspoon of honey
- ¼ cup of almond milk

Instructions

- Take a blender add all the ingredients into a blender and then blend it for 5 minutes

Avocado Coconut Smoothie

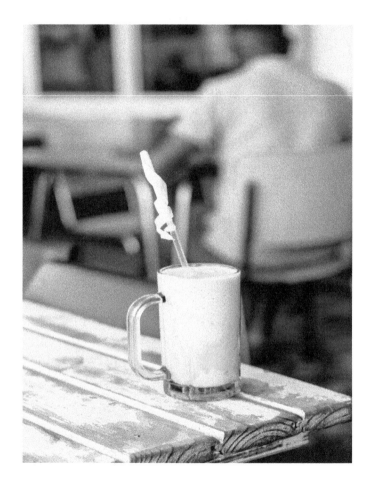

Preparation time: 1-2 minutes
Blending time: 2 minutes
Servings: 2

Ingredients

- 2 cups of avocado
- 1 cup shredded coconut
- ½ cup coconut dairy-free cream
- 1 tsp coconut oil
- Stevia (as per taste)
- Few ice cubes

Instructions

- Blend all these ingredients to make a creamy textured smoothie. Sprinkle shredded coconut on the top after pouring in the glasses.

Cinnamon Smoothie

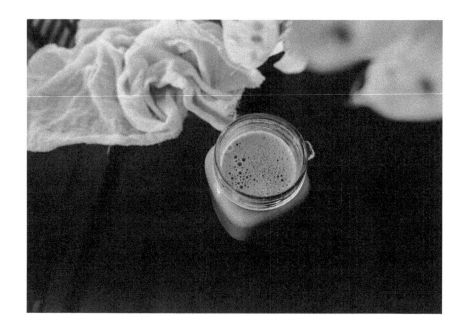

Preparation time: 1-2 minutes
Blending time: 2 minutes
Servings: 2

Ingredients

- ½ tsp cinnamon
- 1 cup almond milk
- 1 cup almond powder
- 1 cup cashew powder
- Few ice cubes
- 1 tbsp peanut butter
- Stevia (as per taste)

Instructions

- With help of the blender, shake all of these ingredients to make the homogeneous smoothie.
- Pour in the glasses and sprinkle cinnamon on them.

Raspberry Avocado Smoothie

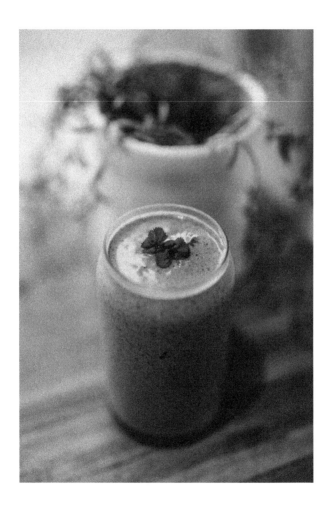

Preparation time: 1-2 minutes
Blending time: 2 minutes
Servings: 2

Ingredients

- 2 cups avocados
- 1 cup frozen raspberries
- 1 cup kale
- Monk fruit (as per your taste)
- Few ice cubes
- 1 tbsp collagen powder
- ½ cup iced water

Instructions

- In the blender, combine and mix all of these ingredients in blending mode. Also, shake at pulse mode to dissolve all the ice. Garnish with raspberries on top.

Keto Pumpkin Smoothie

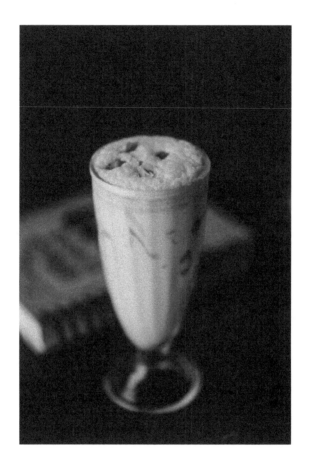

Preparation time: 1-2 minutes
Blending time: 2 minutes
Servings: 2

Ingredients

- 2 cups of pumpkin purée
- ½ cup of greek yogurt
- 1 cup of hazelnuts
- ½ cup almonds
- ½ tsp ginger
- Pinch of salt
- Few ice cubes

Instructions

- Just blend all of these amazing ingredients in the mixer or a juicer. Serve in breakfast with hazelnuts garnished on top.

Green Citrus Smoothie

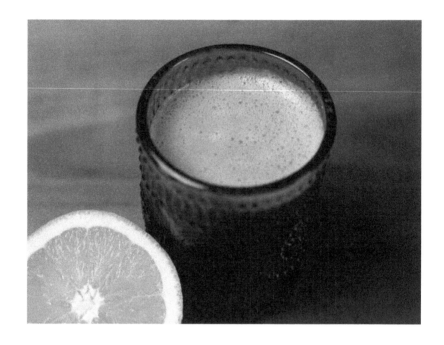

Preparation time: 1-2 minutes
Blending time: 2 minutes
Servings: 2

Ingredients

- 2 tbsp lemon juice (fresh)
- 2 tbsp orange juice (fresh)
- 3 tbsp grapefruit juice (fresh)
- 2 tbsp lime juice (fresh)
- 1 cup kale
- 1 cup zucchini
- Ice cubes
- ½ cup ice cold water

Instructions

- Add all of these healthy ingredients in the blending jar and whirl continuously for 2 minutes at high speed so that everything is converted into tiny granules.

Cinnamon iced Coffee Smoothie

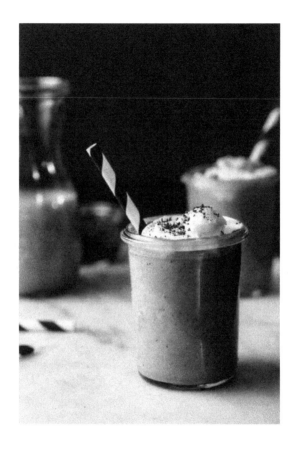

Preparation time: 1-2 minutes
Blending time: 2 minutes
Servings: 2

Ingredients

- ½ tsp bitter coffee
- ½ tsp cocoa (unsweetened)
- ½ tsp cinnamon
- ½ cup dairy-free coconut cream
- 2 tbsp greek yogurt
- 2 cups of ice
- 1 cup almonds (soaked and peeled)
- ½ cup shredded coconut

Instructions

- Take a blender and put all of these ingredients in the blending jar, blend until combined properly.
- In the glasses, add ice cubes or shredded ice and pour this breathtaking smoothie over it.

Pinacolada Smoothie

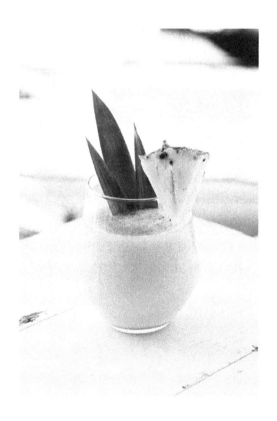

Preparation time: 1-2 minutes
Blending time: 2 minutes
Servings: 2

Ingredients

- 1 cup pineapples
- 1 cup shredded coconut
- 1 cup coconut water (fresh)
- 1 tbsp monk fruit liquid
- 1 cup ice cubes
- 2 tbsp coconut cream (dairy-free)

Instructions

- Put all of these fine ingredients in the blender and blend until all these entities are incorporated within the smoothie.
- Garnish with shredded coconut and serve.

Peach-berry Smoothie

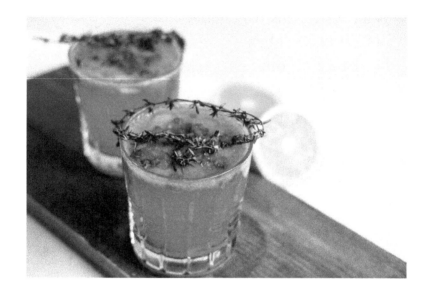

Preparation time: 1-2 minutes
Blending time: 2 minutes
Servings: 2

Ingredients

- 2 cups diced peaches
- 1 cup frozen strawberries
- 1 cup frozen blackberries
- 1 cup frozen raspberries
- 2 tbsp greek yogurt
- 1 cup coconut milk (unsweetened)
- Stevia (as per taste)
- Few ice cubes

Instructions

- Shake these yummy ingredients in the blender at high speed for few seconds to get this extra rich flavored smoothie.

Watermelon rich Chia smoothie

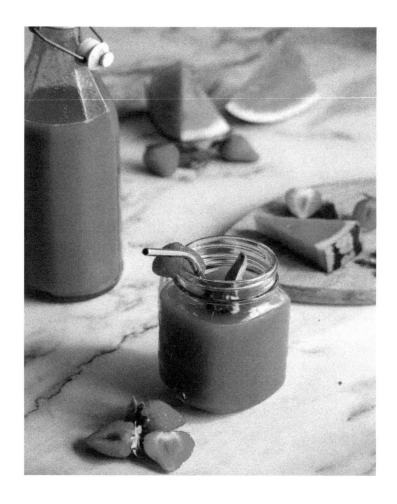

Preparation time: 1-2 minutes
Blending time: 2 minutes
Servings: 2

Ingredients

- 3 cups watermelon (seeds removed)
- 1 cup coconut water
- 1 cup ice cubes
- 1 tbsp chia seeds

Instructions

- Put all of these ingredients in the blender and blend until watermelon is converted into tiny small particles.

Green Detox keto smoothie

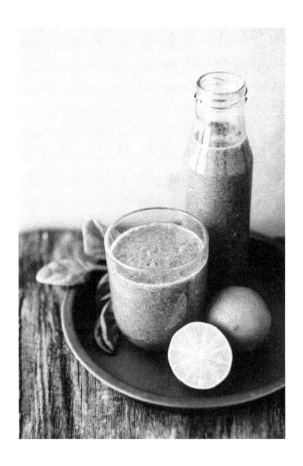

Preparation time: 1-2 minutes
Blending time: 2 minutes
Servings: 2

Ingredients

- 1 cup cucumbers
- 1 cup spinach
- ½ tsp ginger
- Few lemon slices
- 1 tbsp chlorella
- 1 cup ice cubes

Instructions

- Combine all of these ingredients in the electric blender and wait until everything is mixed thoroughly.

Blueberry Coconut Smoothie

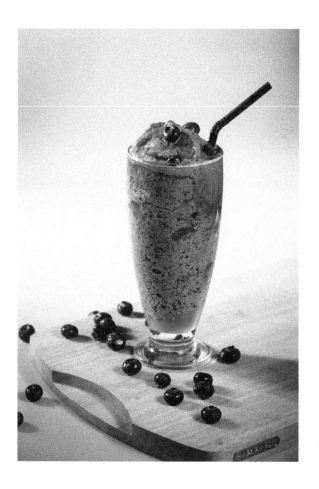

Preparation time: 1-2 minutes
Blending time: 2 minutes
Servings: 2

Ingredients

- 2 cups frozen blueberries
- 1 cup shredded coconut
- 1 cup coconut cream (unsweetened dairy-free)
- 2 tsp monk fruit
- 1 cup ice cubes

Instructions

- Blend all of these healthy ingredients and serve in glasses of your choice.

Vanilla Keto Smoothie

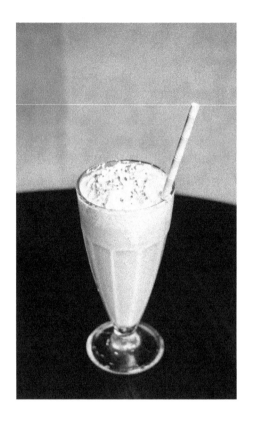

Preparation time: 1-2 minutes
Blending time: 2 minutes
Servings: 1

Ingredients

- 1 cup coconut cream (dairy-free and unsweetened)
- 1 cup walnuts
- 1 tsp vanilla extract
- 1 tbsp collagen powder
- 1 cup ice cubes

Instructions

- Whirl all of these ingredients in the blender until smooth and well mixed.

Keto cranberry Smoothie

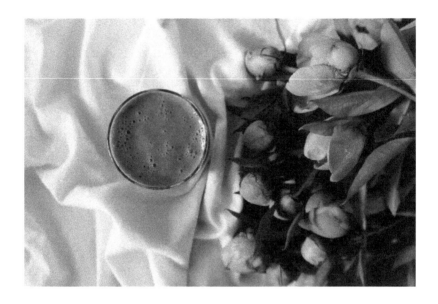

Preparation time: 1-2 minutes
Blending time: 2 minutes
Servings: 2

Ingredients

- 2 cups of frozen cranberries
- 1 cup walnuts
- 1 cup hemp seeds
- 1 cup hemp milk
- 1 cup ice cubes

Instructions

- Put the following entities in the blender and blend until individual constituents are not visible anymore.

Spiced Vanilla Smoothie

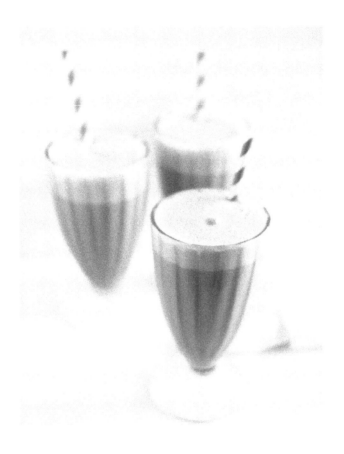

Preparation time: 1-2 minutes
Blending time: 2 minutes
Servings: 2

Ingredients

- 1 cup heavy cream (unsweetened)
- 1 tbsp vanilla protein powder
- 1 tsp vanilla essence
- 1 tsp cinnamon
- 1 tbsp almond powder
- Few ice cubes

Instructions

- Shake all of these mentioned ingredients in the blender, on the pulse, and blending mode to form a rich spiced vanilla smoothie.

Keto Strawberry Banana Smoothie

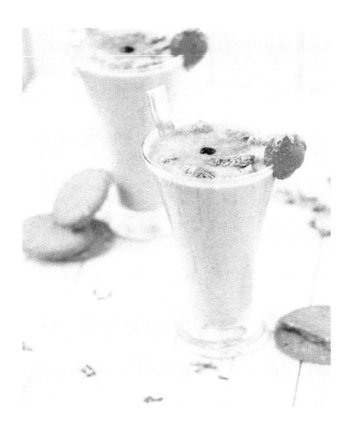

Preparation time: 1-2 minutes
Blending time: 2 minutes
Servings: 2

Ingredients

- 2 cups frozen strawberries
- 1 ripe banana
- ½ tsp vanilla extract
- ½ cup cashew nuts
- ½ cup walnuts
- Few ice cubes
- Monk fruit liquid (as per taste)
- 1 cup hemp milk

Instructions

- Combine all of the above-mentioned ingredients in the blender and whirl until everything is all mixed up and dissolved.

Lime Keto green smoothie

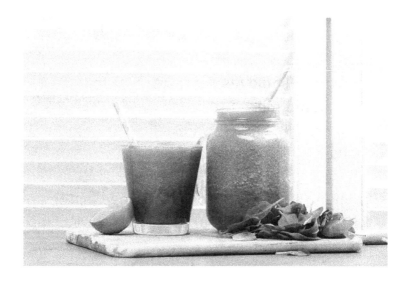

Preparation time: 1-2 minutes
Blending time: 2 minutes
Servings: 2

Ingredients

- 3 tbsp lime juice
- 1 tsp lime zest
- 3-4 lime slices
- 1 cup wheatgrass
- ½ cup iced water
- Few ice cubes

Instructions

- Add all of the following ingredients to the blender and mix them on high speed at blending mode for few seconds or until everything loses its original appearance.
- Put lime slices in glass and then flow the smoothie in those glasses.

Kiwi-berry Smoothie

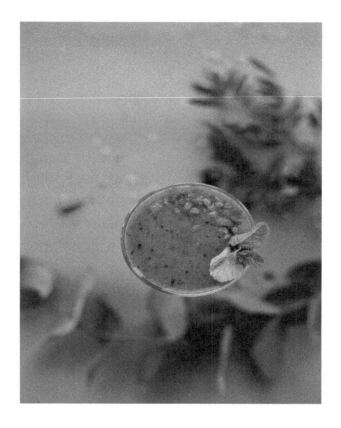

Preparation time: 1-2 minutes
Blending time: 2 minutes
Servings: 2

Ingredients

- 2 cups kiwi cubes
- ½ cup frozen blueberries
- ½ cup frozen raspberries
- 1 cup ice cubes
- 1 tbsp lemon juice
- 1 cup iced water

Instructions

- For making this smoothie, simply put all of these raw ingredients in the blender and wait until they are thoroughly mixed.

Ginger Basil Avocado Smoothie

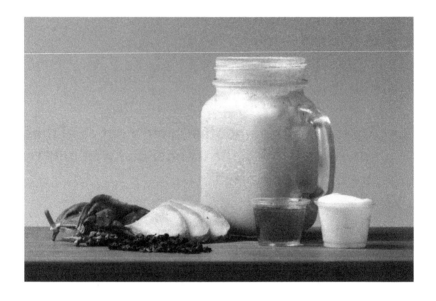

Preparation time: 1-2 minutes
Blending time: 2 minutes
Servings: 2

Ingredients

- 1 cup basil leaves
- 2 cups of avocados
- 1 tsp grated ginger
- 2 tbsp lemon
- Pinch of pink salt
- Few kale leaves
- Few ice cubes
- 1 cup iced water

Instructions

- Just add all of the ingredients that are mentioned above and press the button of the blender and wait until all the constituents lose their visibility.

Blueberry Cauliflower Smoothie

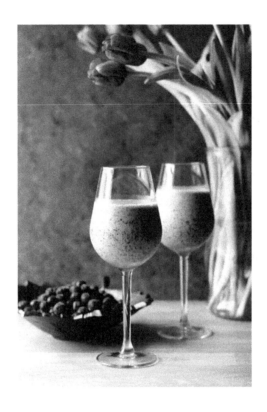

Preparation time: 1-2 minutes
Blending time: 2 minutes
Servings: 2

Ingredients

- 1 cup frozen cauliflower florets
- 1 cup frozen blueberries
- Few mint leaves
- 1 cup almond milk
- Few ice cubes

Instructions

- In the electric blending machine, add these ingredients that are mentioned above and blend. Wait until smooth and uniform. Pour in the glasses and serve.

Blueberry Cheesecake Smoothie

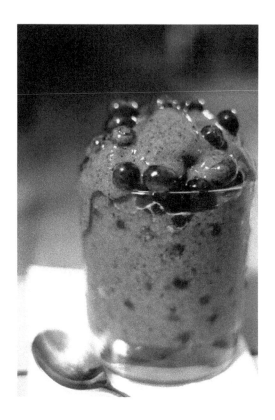

Preparation time: 1-2 minutes
Blending time: 2 minutes
Servings: 2

Ingredients

- 1 cup frozen blueberries
- 1 cup cream cheese (dairy-free & unsweetened)
- ½ cup heavy whipping cream (dairy-free & unsweetened)
- Few ice cubes
- Monk fruit liquid (as per taste)

Instructions

- By using the electric blender, whirl all the ingredients until they are well combined.
- Serve in shake mugs and garnish with blueberries.

Almond Butter Smoothie

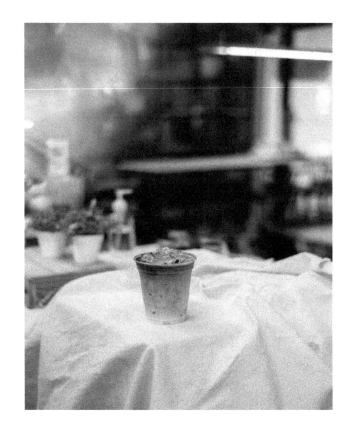

Preparation time: 1-2 minutes
Blending time: 2 minutes
Servings: 2

Ingredients

- 1 cup almonds
- 1 cup coconut cream (dairy-free and unsweetened)
- 1 tbsp almond butter
- 1 tbsp almond-flavored protein powder
- Stevia (according to your taste)
- Few ice cubes

Instructions

- To make this smoothie, add these raw materials mentioned above in the blender and whirl them to get a uniform consistency.

Chocolate Coconut Smoothie

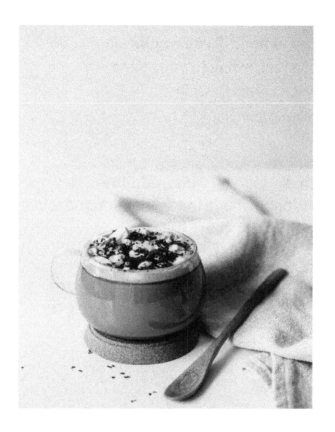

Preparation time: 1-2 minutes
Blending time: 2 minutes
Servings: 2

Ingredients

- 1 tsp unsweetened cocoa
- 1 cup grated coconut
- 1 cup unsweetened coconut cream (dairy-free)
- 1 tbsp collagen powder
- Monk fruit liquid (as per taste)

Instructions

- For making it, put these ingredients in the blender and mix on the pulse mode until well combined.

Chocolate mint Smoothie

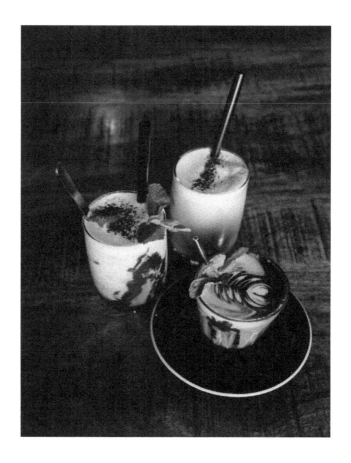

Preparation time: 1-2 minutes
Blending time: 2 minutes
Servings: 2

Ingredients

- 1 cup mint leaves
- 1 tsp unsweetened cocoa
- 1 tbsp cocoa-flavored protein powder
- 1 cup ice cubes
- 1 cup unsweetened cashew milk

Instructions

- Take a blender and put all of these ingredients in it and mix at high speed to get even the consistency of the smoothie.

Choco-spinach Smoothie

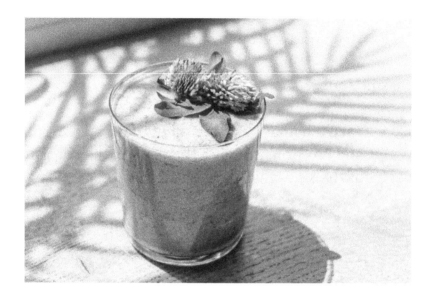

Preparation time: 1-2 minutes
Blending time: 2 minutes
Servings: 2

Ingredients

- 1 tsp dried spinach powder
- 1 tsp cocoa powder
- ½ tsp MCT oil powder
- 1 tbsp unsweetened exogenous ketone base
- 1 tsp coconut butter
- 1 cup heavy cream (unsweetened)

Instructions

- In the electric blender, put in all of the following ingredients and turn it on to make a thick smoothie with everything dissolved in it.

Pumpkin green Smoothie

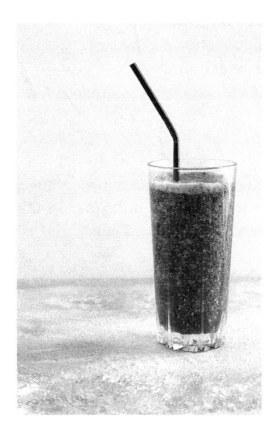

Preparation time: 1-2 minutes
Blending time: 2 minutes
Servings: 2

Ingredients

- 1 cup pumpkin purée
- 1 cup avocados
- 1 cup kale
- 1 cup ice cubes
- 1 cup iced water
- Pinch of salt
- Pinch of ground black pepper

Instructions

- Add pumpkin purée, avocados, kale, ice cubes, and iced water in the blender. Keep it blending until everything is completely mixed up.
- Sprinkle salt and black pepper on it and serve.

Blueberry Walnut Smoothie

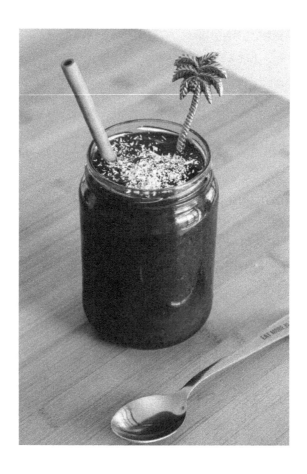

Preparation time: 1-2 minutes
Blending time: 2 minutes
Servings: 2

Ingredients

- 2 cups frozen blueberries
- 1 cup walnuts
- 1 tbsp walnut butter
- 1 cup cashew milk
- 1 tsp MCT oil powder
- Few ice cubes
- 1 tbsp collagen powder

Instructions

- To make this smoothie, add all the raw ingredients to the blender and blend for few seconds until completely mixed. Serve and top with blueberries and walnuts.

Spinach Cucumber Smoothie

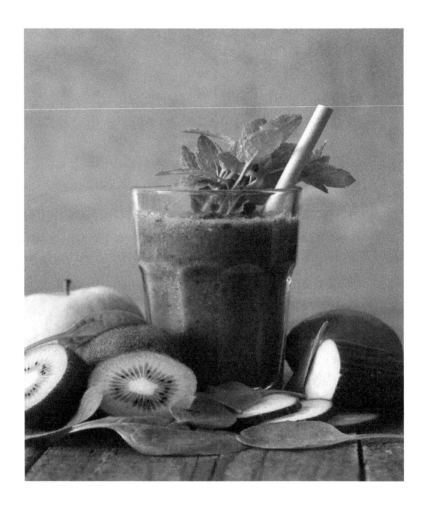

Preparation time: 1-2 minutes
Blending time: 2 minutes
Servings: 2

Ingredients

- 2 cups of spinach
- 1 cup cucumber
- Few orange slices
- 1 cup freshly squeezed orange juice
- Few ice cubes
- 1 tsp flaxseeds

Instructions

- Add all these elements to the blender and mix them until everything is combined very well.
- Pour in the glasses with orange slices in them.

Blueberry Avocado Smoothie

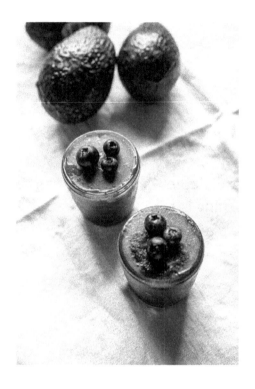

Preparation time: 1-2 minutes
Blending time: 2 minutes
Servings: 2

Ingredients

- 1 cup frozen blueberries
- 2 cups of avocados
- 1 cup ice cubes
- Stevia (as per taste)
- 1 cup unsweetened heavy cream

Instructions

- Mix all these ingredients in the blender until everything is well combined. Garnish with blueberries on top.

Dragonfruit-Watermelon Smoothie

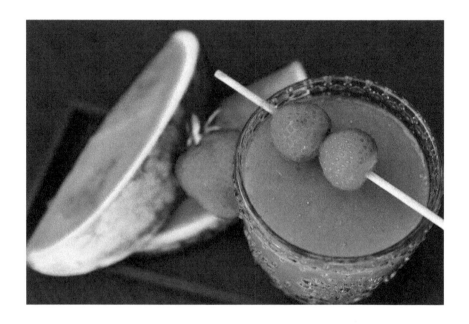

Preparation time: 1-2 minutes
Blending time: 2 minutes
Servings: 2

Ingredients

- 1 cup of dragonfruit cubes
- 2 cups of watermelon cubes
- 1 tsp dragonfruit powder
- 1 tsp lemon zest
- Few ice cubes
- 1 cup iced water

Instructions

- Combine all these ingredients in the blender and serve in the glasses.

Pink Peach Smoothie

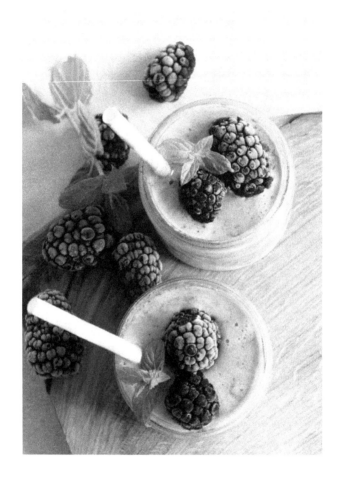

Preparation time: 1-2 minutes
Blending time: 2 minutes
Servings: 2

Ingredients

- 1 tbsp dragonfruit powder
- 2 cups of peaches
- 1 tbsp collagen powder
- 3 tbsp greek yogurt
- Few ice cubes
- ½ cup blackberries for garnishing

Instructions

- Whirl the following ingredients in the blender. When everything combines well, pour them into the glasses.

Pumpkin Spice Smoothie

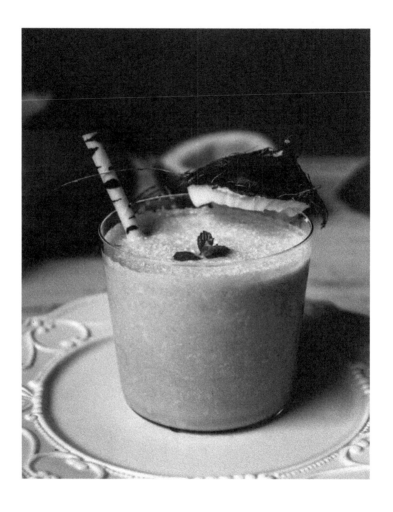

Preparation time: 1-2 minutes
Blending time: 2 minutes
Servings: 2

Ingredients

- 2 cups pumpkin purée
- ½ tsp pumpkin pie spice
- 1 cup heavy cream (unsweetened)
- Monk fruit liquid (as per taste)
- ½ tsp cinnamon powder

Instructions

- Combine all of the following ingredients in the blender. Pour in the glasses and enjoy.

Orange Avocado Smoothie

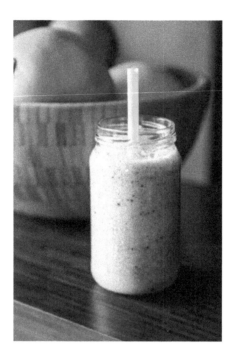

Preparation time: 1-2 minutes
Blending time: 2 minutes
Servings: 2

Ingredients

- 3 cups of avocados
- 2 cups of fresh orange juice
- 1 tsp orange zest
- 12 mint leaves

Instructions

- Mix all the following ingredients in the blender and keep on blending until everything is all mixed up.

Strawberry Zucchini Smoothie

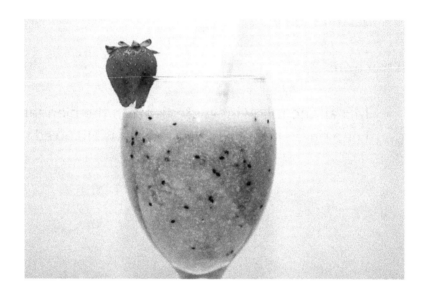

Preparation time: 1-2 minutes
Blending time: 2 minutes
Servings: 2

Ingredients

- 2 cups of strawberries
- 1 cup of zucchini
- 1 cup coconut water
- Few ice cubes

Instructions

- Grind all these components in the blender until a well-combined mixture is obtained.

Coconut-Blackberry Mint Smoothie

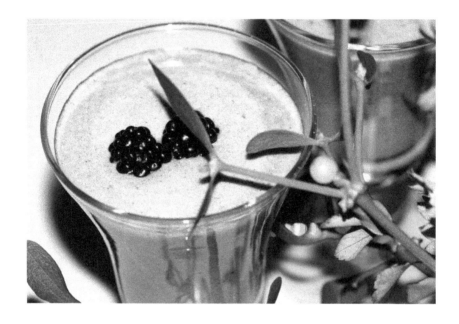

Preparation time: 1-2 minutes
Blending time: 2 minutes
Servings: 2

Ingredients

- 2 cups of blackberries
- 1 cup shredded coconut
- 1 cup mint leaves
- 1 cup ice cubes
- 1 cup coconut water
- Pinch of salt
- Pinch of paper

Instructions

- Put the following ingredients in the mixing blender. Blend until smooth. Stream into the glasses and serve.

Cinnamon Cream Strawberry Smoothie

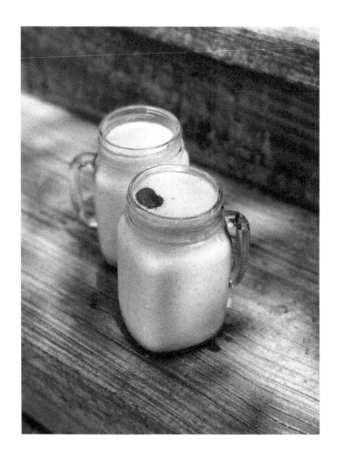

Preparation time: 1-2 minutes
Blending time: 2 minutes
Servings: 2

Ingredients

- 1 cup heavy unsweetened cream
- ½ tsp cinnamon
- 2 cups of strawberries
- 1 tsp chia seeds
- 1 tsp exogenous ketone base
- Few ice cubes
- 1 tsp NutraSweet

Instructions

- For making it, put these ingredients in the blender and mix on the pulse mode until well combined.

Chocolate Cauliflower Smoothie

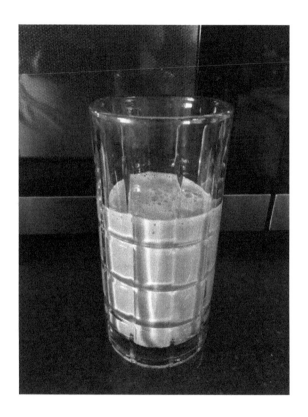

Preparation time: 1-2 minutes
Blending time: 2 minutes
Servings: 2

Ingredients

- 1 tsp unsweetened cocoa
- 2 cups of frozen cauliflower florets
- 1 tbsp chocolate-flavored protein powder
- 1 cup unsweetened heavy cream
- Few ice cubes

Instructions

- Blend the following ingredients in the blender until all of the components are fully combined. Serve in shake mugs.

Coconut Vanilla Smoothie

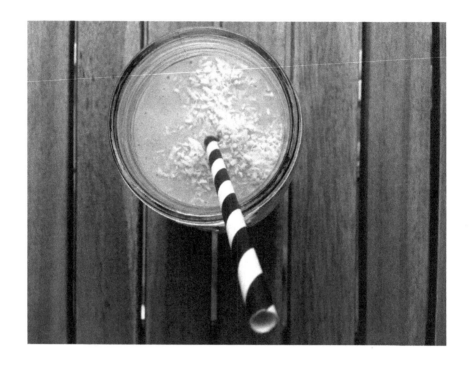

Preparation time: 1-2 minutes
Blending time: 2 minutes
Servings: 2

Ingredients

- 1 cup unsweetened coconut cream
- 1 tsp vanilla essence
- 1 cup shredded coconut
- 3 tbsp coconut water
- 1 tbsp vanilla flavored protein powder
- Few ice cubes

Instructions

- Blend all of the ingredients to form a uniform, thick consistency. Stream in the glasses and serve.

Starfruit Lettuce Smoothie

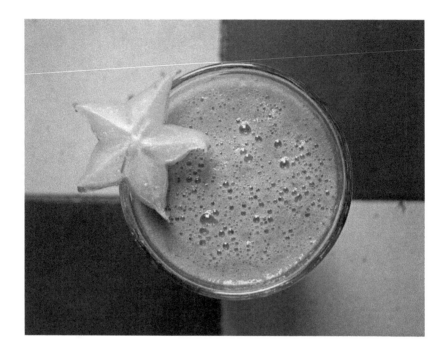

Preparation time: 1-2 minutes
Blending time: 2 minutes
Servings: 2

Ingredients

- 1 cup diced starfruit
- 2 cups Roman lettuce
- 2 tbsp lemon juice
- ½ cup basil leaves
- 1 cup ice cubes
- 1 cup iced water

Instructions

- To make this smoothie, combine all of these substances in the blending machine and swirl until mixed.

Coffee Cashew Smoothie

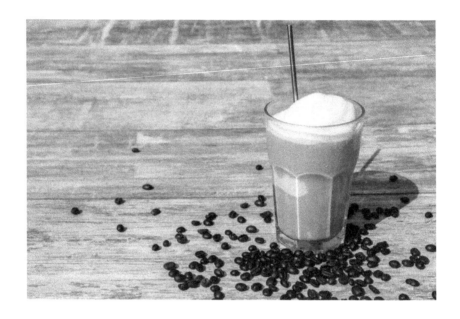

Preparation time: 1-2 minutes
Blending time: 2 minutes
Servings: 2

Ingredients

- 1 tbsp cashew butter
- 1 cup cashew nuts
- 1 tsp coffee powder
- 1 cup cashew milk
- 1 tbsp coffee-flavored protein powder
- Few ice cubes

Instructions

- In the blender, put all the substances and blend them to form the smoothie.
- Pour in the glasses and serve.

Avocado-Nut milk Smoothie

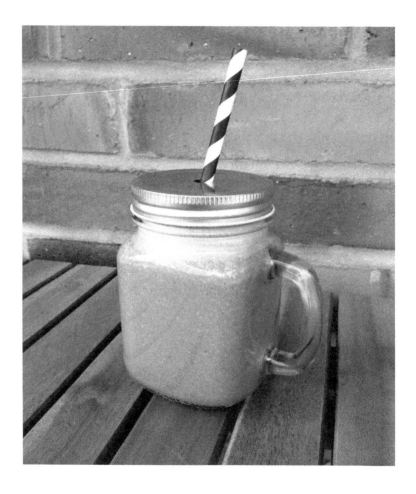

Preparation time: 1-2 minutes
Blending time: 2 minutes
Servings: 2

Ingredients

- 2 cups of avocados
- 1 cup nut milk
- 1 tbsp chia seeds
- Stevia (as per taste)

Instructions

- Blend avocados, nut milk, chia seeds, and stevia and serve.

Tomato green Smoothie

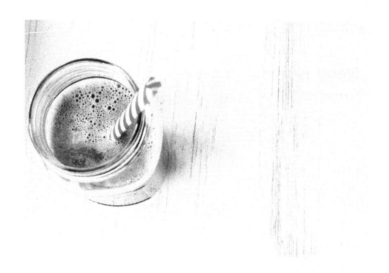

Preparation time: 1-2 minutes
Blending time: 2 minutes
Servings: 2

Ingredients

- 2 cup tomatoes
- 1 cup parsley
- 1 cup celery
- 2 tbsp lime juice
- Few ice cubes
- 1/2 cup iced water

Instructions

- Put the above ingredients in the blender and turn on the blending mode. Wait until everything gets mixed up.

Ginger Spirulina Detox Smoothie

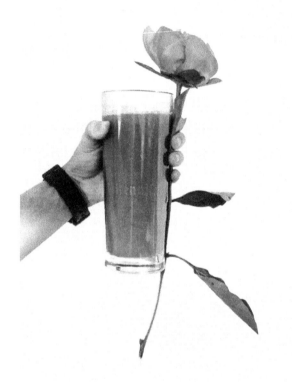

Preparation time: 1-2 minutes
Blending time: 2 minutes
Servings: 2

Ingredients

- ½ tsp fresh ginger paste
- 1 tbsp Spirulina powder
- 2 cups celery
- ½ cup cucumbers
- 12 mint leaves

Instructions

- Make the smoothie by blending all of these ingredients.
- Pour in the glasses and enjoy your keto diet.

Lemon Turmeric Smoothie

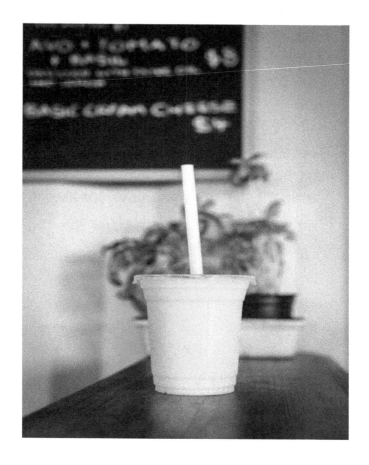

Preparation time: 1-2 minutes
Blending time: 2 minutes
Servings: 2

Ingredients

- 4-5 lemon slices
- 3 tbsp lemon juice
- ½ tsp turmeric
- 3 tbsp greek yogurt
- Few ice cubes
- 1 tsp spinach powder
- ½ cup water

Instructions

- Put lemon juice, turmeric, greek yogurt, ice cubes, spinach powder, and water in the blending jar and blend until every component is mixed.
- Put in some lemon slices in the glasses and stream the smoothie in the glasses.

Pear Strawberry Smoothie

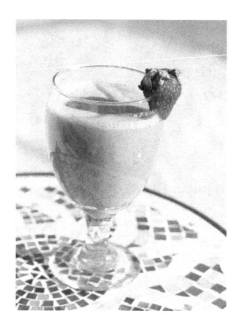

Preparation time: 1-2 minutes
Blending time: 2 minutes
Servings: 2

Ingredients

- 2 cups diced pears
- 1 cup frozen strawberries
- ½ cup heavy unsweetened cream
- ½ cup hemp milk
- 1 tsp almond butter
- Few ice cubes

Instructions

- Blend all of these at high speed until each particle turns very tiny. Serve in your favourite glasses.

Strawberry Ginger Smoothie

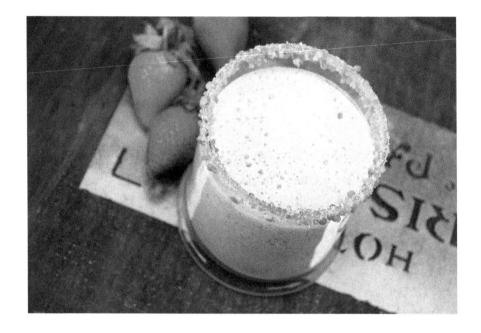

Preparation time: 1-2 minutes
Blending time: 2 minutes
Servings: 2

Ingredients

- 2 cups frozen strawberries
- ½ tsp fresh ginger paste
- 1 cup coconut milk
- 1 tsp coconut oil
- 1 tbsp collagen powder
- ¼ tsp cinnamon powder
- Few ice cubes

Instructions

- In order to make smoothie, and blend all of these at high speed till they are well combined or converted into unrecognizable particles. Serve in the smoothie jars.

Kale Berry Smoothie

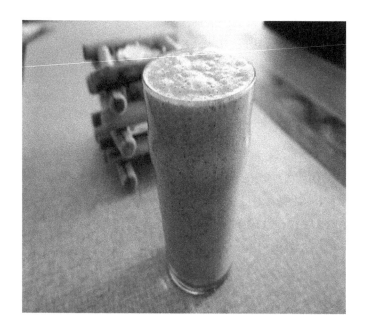

Preparation time: 1-2 minutes
Blending time: 2 minutes
Servings: 2

Ingredients

- 2 cups kale
- 1 cup strawberries
- 1 cup greek yogurt
- Pinch of salt
- Few ice cubes

Instructions

- Blend all of these at high speed and serve in the smoothie jars.

Salted Sugar-free caramel smoothie

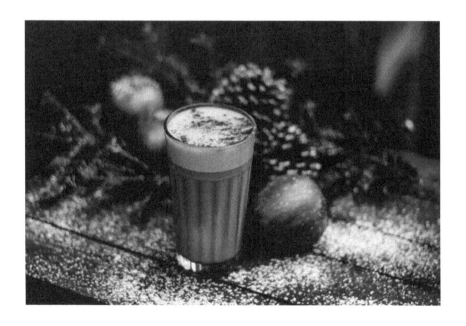

Preparation time: 1-2 minutes
Blending time: 2 minutes
Servings: 2

Ingredients

- ¼ tsp salt
- Few ice cubes
- 1 cup heavy unsweetened cream
- 2 tbsp caramel flavored protein powder
- 1 tbsp almond powder
- ½ tbsp cinnamon powder

Instructions

- Add all of these elements to the blender and mix them very well at high speed to dissolve all the powder and ice lumps.

Green Papaya Smoothie

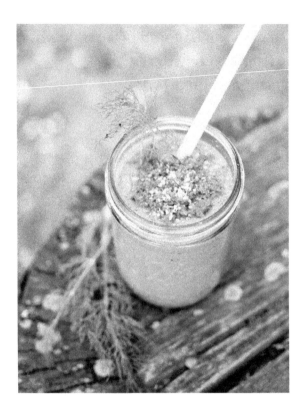

Preparation time: 1-2 minutes
Blending time: 2 minutes
Servings: 2

Ingredients

- 2 cups of diced papaya
- 1 cup roman lettuce
- 12 mint leaves
- 1 cup ice cubes
- 1 cup iced water

Instructions

- Put the following elements in the blender and keep them blending until they are converted into very tiny particles.

Grapefruit Pumpkin Smoothie

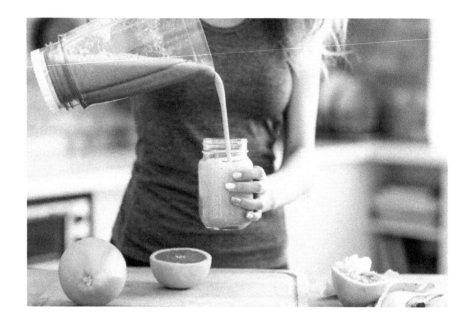

Preparation time: 1-2 minutes
Blending time: 2 minutes
Servings: 2

Ingredients

- 1 cup freshly squeezed grapefruit juice
- 1 tsp grapefruit zest
- 1 cup spinach
- 1 cup pumpkin purée
- Few ice cubes

Instructions

- By using the blender put all these ingredients and swirl them when everything is equally dispersed in the smoothie.

Lemon Rosewater Smoothie

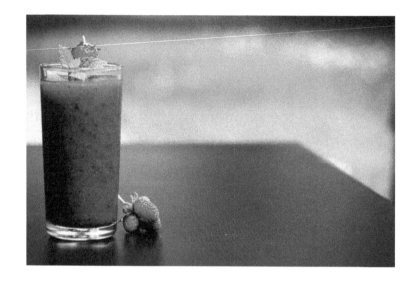

Preparation time: 1-2 minutes
Blending time: 2 minutes
Servings: 2

Ingredients

- 2 cups frozen strawberries
- 1 tbsp lemon juice
- ½ tsp lemon zest
- ¼ tsp rose water
- ½ cup iced water
- 1 cup shredded ice

Instructions

- With the help of blender put all of these elements and mix until it turns homogeneous.
- Pour in the smoothie jars and serve.